Hair Down to There

Hair Down to There

Dr. Chandris McCoy, BND

Copyright © 2012 by Dr. Chandris McCoy, BND.

Library of Congress Control Number: 2012917803
ISBN: Hardcover   978-1-4797-2251-8
               Softcover   978-1-4797-2250-1
               Ebook   978-1-4797-2252-5

All rights reserved. No part of this book may be reproduced or transmitted in any form or by any means, electronic or mechanical, including photocopying, recording, or by any information storage and retrieval system, without permission in writing from the copyright owner.

By no means is this book intended to be one that offers cures or remedies for hair problems. This is not an exhaustive work about black hair due to the variations among black hair. In essence this work is done from a naturopathic position addressing commonalities in the experiences of black women and their hair. This is not a medical work. It will not diagnose or treat hair conditions. It serves to educate, suggest, and inform readers of hair care options.

This book was printed in the United States of America.

To order additional copies of this book, contact:
Xlibris Corporation
1-888-795-4274
www.Xlibris.com
Orders@Xlibris.com
118603

Contents

This book is dedicated to My Heavenly Father who created my genes, to my parents Curtis Chaney and Ethel Edwards who gave me my genes, to my grandparents Leroy and Norma Logan who gave my genes a home and a heritage.

Foreword

by Matthew W. Brown, MD

I had the pleasure of first meeting Dr. Chandris McCoy when I was in the seventh grade and she was in the eighth. She made an impression. It was at an all-region band concert, where East Texas middle schools sent their most talented musicians to play a concert they learned earlier that afternoon. I am sure the sound was less than melodic. Chandris and I also played saxophone, and while I don't remember which chair I rated, I do recall that she was rated higher than me and sat to my left. I also recall that while most of the young musicians were wearing the equivalent of khakis or Sunday clothes, the young black woman to my left was wearing a long silvery blue shimmering gown and had long smooth, straight hair. She was tall. She was stunning.

There were many people of color in my high school, but only a handful shared my advanced gifted and honors classes, and only one of those students rode my bus, Chandris. Our paths had crossed again as different middle schools funnel into the same high school. Her family had moved to the south side of town, and we then rode the same bus home and became fast friends. Dr. McCoy had long smooth, straight hair the entire time, even as a premed student in liberal Austin, Texas.

I have an autosomal dominant gene for premature gray hair. My hair started to change colors at age sixteen and was noticeably different by the time I was in college. I never colored my hair partly because I thought it was unique and most of my friends knew I had gray hair and would then know I was just coloring my natural hair. I never thought about this being an advantage or disadvantage; it was just hair. Until I was in medical school. As a student, I would enter a patient's room with the staff surgeon to talk about their medical condition. The patients would direct their questions to me and ask me what they should do, despite the fact that my instructing surgeon was standing next to me. My silver hair had falsely implied experience and wisdom. I was careful not to take advantage of this misperception but appreciated the confidence my hair instilled when I had the knowledge and skills to back it up.

It is interesting to ponder the beauty regime that was set in place by Chandris's grandmother. The advantages of straightened hair, both perceived and real, she imparted and the consequential personal struggle of altering one's own natural, God-given tresses. Certainly all God's plan in action.

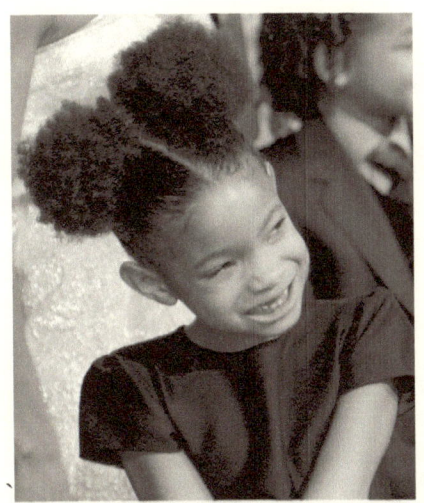
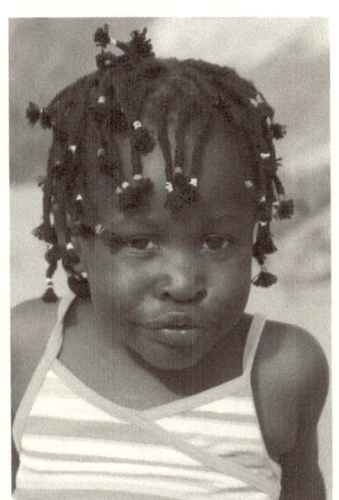
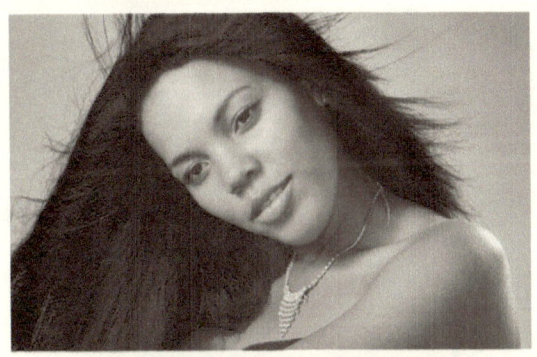
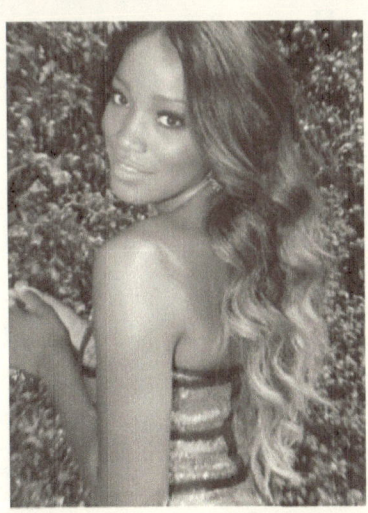

Introduction

There are many reasons for this book, but only a few will be mentioned. There are myths concerning Black hair that must be silenced. Mainstream editors do not address the beauty challenges of Black hair in proportion to the numbers of Black readers. The dynamics of Black hair are not brought to the forefront enough that we might better appreciate and understand the multicultural world in which we live.

This book does not exist to magnify any schism within the Black race (class, religion, socioeconomics, etc.). It does not exist to increase any misgivings between races. It simply tells of a common experience that many Black women have. It specifically speaks to those desiring longer hair. There is encouragement for those women to embrace what God has given them.

CHAPTER 1

A Hidden Glamour

Cutie

Yes, I am a cutie
Since you have been working double duty

First you straighten me
Then you curl me
Kinda confusing
'Twas not my choosing

A made-up mind
I'd never expect
Afros, braids, waves
And you still ain't through with me yet!

Every little girl wants long hair, or at least that was my impression decades ago. Most of the television shows and magazine covers that I saw had pictures of women with long flowing hair. They never showed me the glamour of short Black hair. I even wondered where the glamour of Black hair had been placed. So many Black women in my life had instances when they felt they were considered second best by their contemporaries because of their hair length or type. This is known because of my observance of the maltreatment of others. Also within those years is remembered the ridicule from those who did not approve the diversity of Black hair regarding its length or texture. The saddest truth is that the humor stemmed from a culture not different from the Black culture. But it is propagated by those with similar hair, skin type, and culture of Black people.

Bare

It's neither here nor there
Why do I care
After ridicule while in school
I wish my head were bare

Who Taught You?

If you hate me
You won't date me
You won't waste my time
A man unpleased from my head to my knees
Is really no man of mine

Used to play together
Walk home in all kinds of weather
We marched to ensure our kids' liberty
The harsh words spoken make no sense to me

Bald head, chicken head, nappy too
Are just to name a few
Of all the people who could have berated me
It had to be you?

What happened to make you so ashamed?
What happened in your youth
Please tell me the truth

I always had dark eyes
My curls are no surprise
Are you my enemy in disguise?

Who taught you to hate
Who taught you the
Best hair is straight?

This reality of disapproval and insecurity somewhat propels the multibillion-dollar revenue of the Black hair industry. Whether it is a hairpiece or a wig, the markets have profited from the personal dissatisfaction of many women. They have yet to match their earnings with helping consumers to embrace individuality.

This book includes poems and prayers that address the pain and anger that has been left to a community of women because of their hair type. This community is not located on a map, but it still exists. They live in a rejected and lonely place. At times there is anger and resentment in this place. This community may frequent your grocery stores or your shopping malls. Usually they are silent about this harsh reality, but now is the time to speak up regardless of the backlash. The inclusion of prayers serves only to urge people to forgive, encourage apology, and others to happily repent. The voices of such treatment have been squelched by convenience and personal denial. A hairdressing or hair appointment does not erase the unjust partiality or sensitize society of the sadness endured by the hearts of others. No longer should we hide the experiences about Black women and their hair. But it is due time to sensitize society about the challenges that some Black women have had simply over hair. Also, this effort to encourage others to think about how they treat Black girls and women will truly yield more benefit than silence will.

Black Is Beautiful

Like all hair
My hair is sometimes dutiful
Till death do we part
I do love it with all my heart

I love the way I can tell
If a man is a lover of his own curl
When I don my natural curls
Just to see if he knows

That I will embrace them
Whether he stays or whether he goes

From Crystal Gayle to my English teacher, I was assured that long hair was just a matter of time because we all were females. I had no understanding of just how much heredity and lifestyle make a difference in the hair I have. Now I don't waste time in ignorance wishing for something that my genes will not produce.

Wasted Praise

Hair, hair, you are the epitome of unfair
I wish I did not care
Not to mention
You get ridiculous attention

Just to let me down on rainy days
Talk about wasted praise!

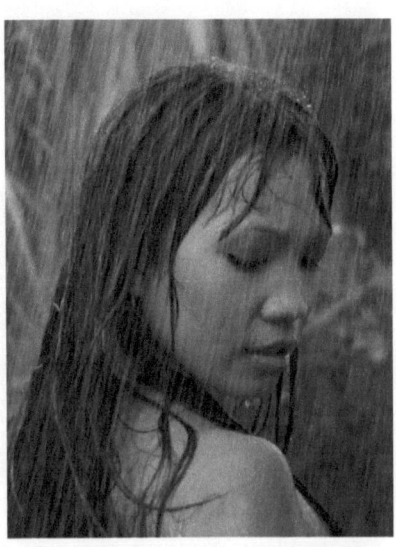

Over time I thought of my hair as a taskmaster of sorts without wondering why it was so important to my grandma that any semblance of Afrocentricity was unacceptable to her. I never even thought to ask her about it. I only knew that it was understood that since I lived in my grandparents' house, I had to like whatever they liked regardless of the cost to my understanding of self-love. I truly could not reconcile the logic behind washing my hair and complimenting my curls immediately before they met Grandma's hot straightening comb. Big thick locks were always victorious over me in that I never had it my way, which would have been easier and painless. Grimacing in a chair with heat and more heat was part of my cost for beauty at a young age, and many other little girls across the nation paid it as well the very same way.

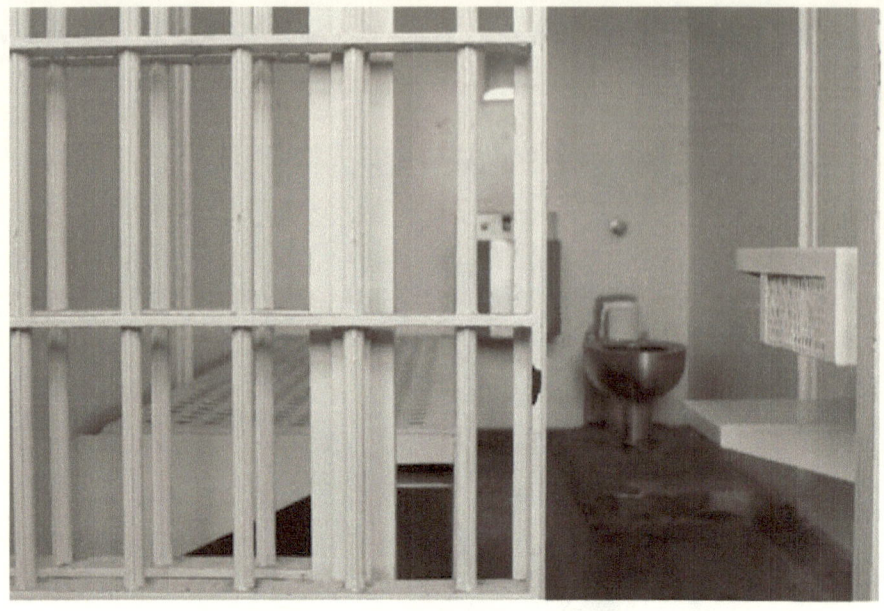

Mama's Crime

Mama's crime was not silent or even sublime
She brought me here yet she taught me dear
To secretly and silently dislike these fluffy curls of mine

How could she say "Black is beautiful"?
Made this girl feel like combing hair was too dutiful
Calling it out of its name
Made God's creation feel ashamed

She did not kill, but stole my self-esteem
So many other girls withstood the very same thing
But freely she walks every day
And I know her mom did her the same way

The following compliments after my hairdressing were due me since I quietly sat while having my image transformed. I grew to like the way I looked. It was the only look I knew about, actually. No matter the cost to my understanding of God's divine purpose for my image. I simply thought that if my family liked it, then I liked it too. What was a matter of time was my understanding that my hair length and thickness was God's choice and not mine. So over the years, I learned a few untruths about hair as I lived the reality of how to deal with a head full of hair. One question, however, seemed to remain with me whether I wore braids or straightened hair.

My pressing question was this: where are the Black women with long flowing hair? I understood that my geographical location had little to do with my lack of observing long hair. Knowledge of cultural differences did not answer my question. All of my great-aunts with the long locks had cut their hair by the time I was born. I could find no books at my public library that would address the question. No magazines seemed abreast of my dilemma about hair. Apparently, Black hair was not important to the editors of the magazines, but it was important to me. I did not ask this question verbally for fear of being rebuked and maligned. Conversations with my cosmetologist Aunt Cindy shed much light on the matter. I will shed light on the matter as well in this book.

One day while she was studying hair, I grabbed her main textbook. In it were terms I could not pronounce, but the pictures were very helpful. I read and saw that Asians had the straightest hair, not white Americans. This was the beginning of my understanding about hair!

Do They Love God?

I do not get it
Maybe I should
Just quit this
You know, being a fake-haired one

First they call it nappy
How am I supposed to be happy
Then they say, "God loves me"
Sure *He* loves me

But me they can see
So how can they say they love God
The simple things in life
Are really not that hard

Why did He give me such stubborn hair
I place my curls right here
But they opt to go over there

The truth of it all?
At least I have hair to compare

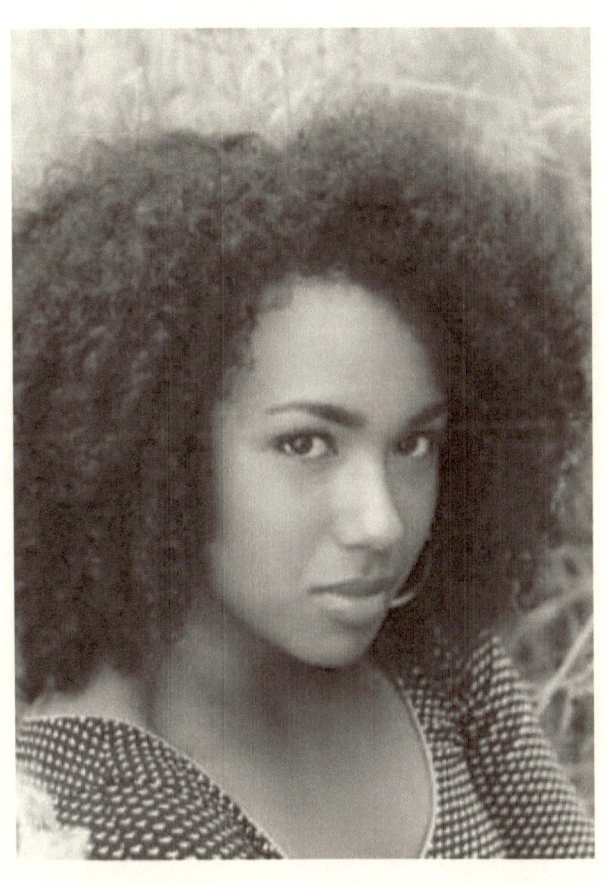

CHAPTER 2

But Your Hair Is Different

My first experience with love was within the context of the Logan family. This family was as solid as solid could be, or so I understood. We held everything in common, and whatever differences we may have had did not matter to us too much.

My Aunt Barbara was not a cosmetologist, yet she had an artist's eye. She also won my heart on many matters because of her intelligence. So when she told me that she would not benefit the same way I would when using specific hair care products, I was perplexed. After all, we both are Black. She taught me that we had different parents, and that made our hair look and feel slightly different. Aunt Barbara's hair was more predisposed to tangles than mine. My outlook on Black hair since then has never been the same. Telling me that my hair was different from hers was both bittersweet. I felt like we were the same even down to the root, but we were not.

Why is hair even an issue within the Black community? This I learned at first in the presence of my Aunt Jackie and later in the presence of women who interfaced with me to compliment me on my hair. The reason is historical. Slaves were pitted against each other to ensure the solidarity of the institution of slavery according to the historical Willie Lynch letter of 1712.

One tool that was used was what involuntary miscegenation produced. Blacks with the lightest skin or straightest hair were often favored or pulled off the fields to work inside the slave masters' houses. Such activity caused the remaining slaves to resent the house slaves' advantages and the slaves themselves. Such lack of unity gave the slave masters comfort. They knew that the success of any revolt required unity. They knew that a chance of togetherness among slaves was slim. This resentment decreased the chance of a slave's united front against the master.

Yesteryear's partiality that haunts and taunts Black people (including children) today has caused some people to embrace such behavior at the expense of others' self-esteem. Partiality is often witnessed toward the person with the head that is full of flowing wavy or straight or relaxed locks within the Black culture. Therefore, it is imperative that we must understand the ramifications behind hair that are both physical and spiritual.

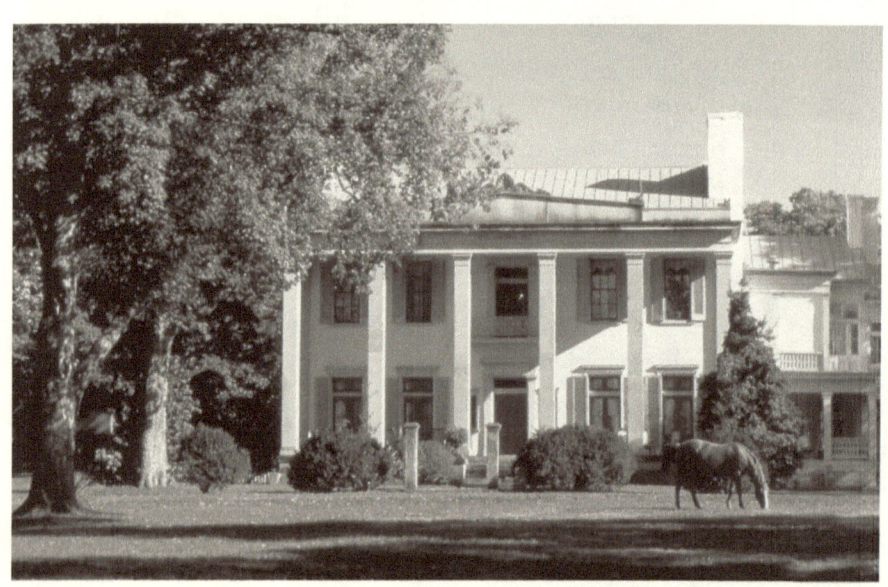

Sister

Regardless of what they shout
Whether I have that hair or not
Grade is not what sisterhood is about
You may have the softer and longer tresses
But humility is what God blesses

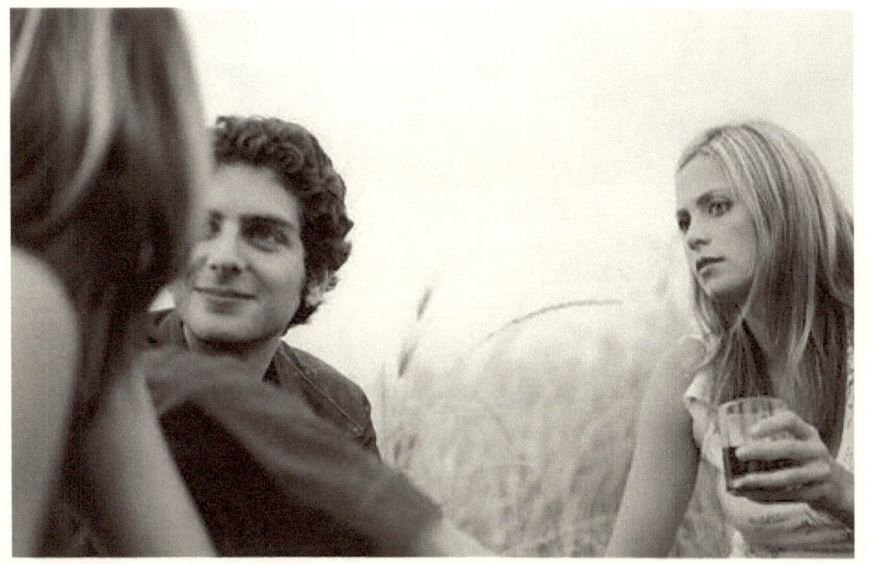

Jealousy

What have you done for me?
Used to have a lot of friends
Now I have only three

When we came over on the ship
Over hair did we trip?

Or is it just now that we cry
Is it just now that we vie?
Over length and curls
Over being the cutest of all the girls?

Jealousy, you took love out of life's equation
You added evil to my frustration
Mind you I am the one steering this ship
And I am so hating *this* trip

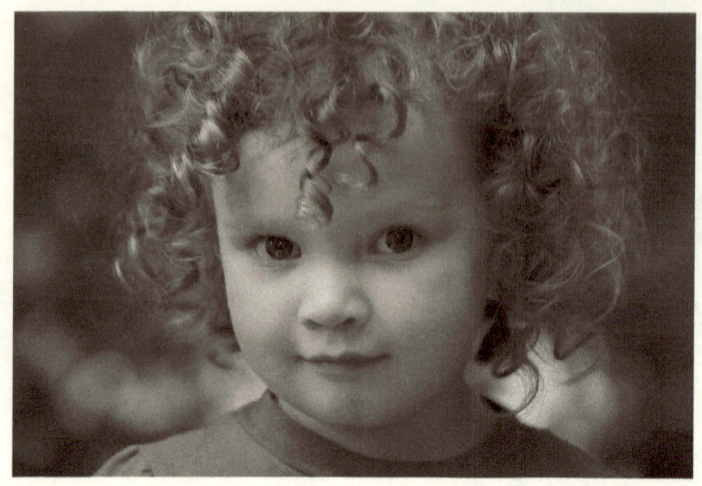

People Pleaser

One, two, three
Why she holla at me?
I did nothin' wrong
My hair is just too strong

Mother calls it rough,
But I call it tough
To get through
Unkind and negative stuff

Jesus, please deliver me
From the chair of hypocrisy
Help me to love your creativity

'Cause 4, 5, 6
My mom is full of tricks
As she approaches the church and steeple
Nubian princess puts up her façade
To successfully please all people

7, 8, 9
Every Sunday is less than Divine
As others like her tell me good-bye
I wonder so quietly if they also make their pretty
Girls cry

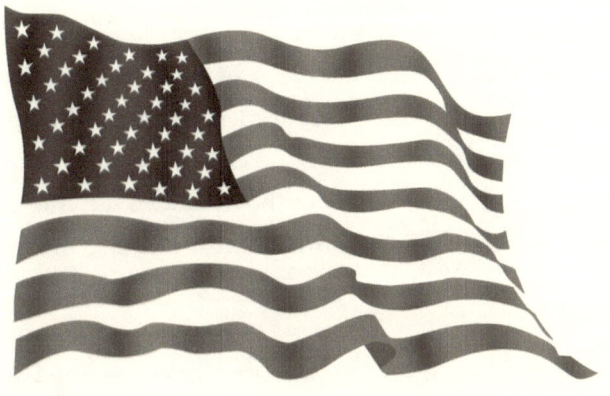

Mama Said

Mama said nice fine hair means
Someone else was there
Not necessarily that they cared

So what about the kinky stuff?
People may pass you over
Some quietly think it's too rough
But remember rough rhymes with tough

It symbolizes what we had to be
To leave our homes involuntarily
To fight for true liberty
To remain and procreate

To successfully love instead of hate
To remember the One who loves you
Those beautiful curls He did create
To love them too is awesome and great

When asked what hair is, one is able to get a number of responses to describe the same thing. A medical doctor would answer differently from a fifth grader who would also answer differently from a zoologist. No matter who you ask, it is a symbol of femininity that girls just can't do without. Hair may be the reason one child was favored over the other or why one person landed a job or boyfriend over the other person. Whatever the case, the ramifications behind hair are unmistakable and memorable.

In addition to this observation, some have suffered injury due to their hair's length or texture. Some have suffered ostracism. Examples of ostracism may include being left out of a crowd of girls who gather to laugh at the child in question and also being left out of a lunchtime gathering. It is true that these examples are simple, but the memories of being left out of a crowd do still poke at the victim. Because of this, forgiveness must be featured. The most important thing concerning any kind of injury is forgiveness. This is where hair can have a spiritual aspect. Regardless of the details of the hurt, one must forgive the instigator. This is to ensure spiritual progression (Mark 11:26). When we refuse to forgive, we are placed on the losing side by default. No follicle is worth my personal advance. How about yours? Honestly, you may think you are saved, but if the Lord can forgive your sins, then there is no doubt that you can forgive someone else's offense toward you. Just remember Jesus forgave *while* He was being crucified. He did not just wait until the pain stopped. If you think that it is not probable or possible, then ask the Lord to help you in this matter. I would not spend time writing on forgiveness if unforgiveness had no eternal consequences. But it does. After all, why would God forgive you if you do not forgive others? Therefore, do not you deserve to go on with life? God will not acknowledge our prayers without forgiveness. Therefore, it only makes sense to forgive others and proceed with life.

Autoimmunity in Your Community

Is autoimmunity in your community?
Is it shrouded as a smile?
But in actuality is jealousy

When you look at me
Why don't you see thee?
We are quite common indeed
Whether in dreads or beads
Your hair is quite beautiful you see
There really is no need to be catty towards me

You must recognize your sister and brother
That they will not be harmed by the words of another
That they will do no harm to someone's heart
Can't you see how ignorance
tears us apart

How will we live?
How will we grow?
Amidst autoimmunity, only God knows

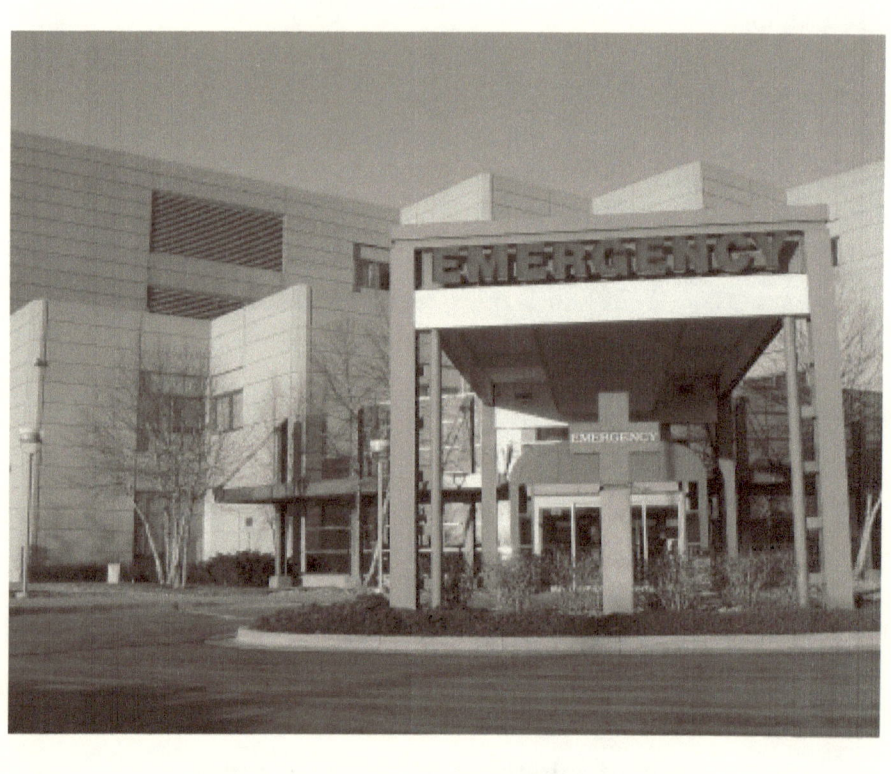

CHAPTER 3

I Found "There"

I learned at a tender age that having long braids gave me favor that I did not necessarily earn. Little did I know that hours of sitting still at the hands of a skilled beautician would be followed with gazes of adoration for the meticulous handiwork of the stylist. Braids are such a beautiful way to wear natural hair. Nonetheless, I yearned to know how to make my hair grow down to there as usual.

So where is "there"? My personal quest for this "there" started years before synthetic hair was worn by the masses. By observing the smiles of others who had simply added hair extensions, something became clear to me. Those women with new hair had discovered "there" while looking at themselves and the smiles of approval of their friends and even strangers.

"There" is not a place that can be located on every woman or girl, but it is a place of acceptance and approval sometimes laced with accolade. It is at the discretion of each female's taste. It is no doubt that "there" is a matter of necessity. It is needed that one is content with one's own appearance regardless of the opinions of others. The Psalmist gives us a great example of this when he writes that I am fearfully and wonderfully made (Ps. 139).

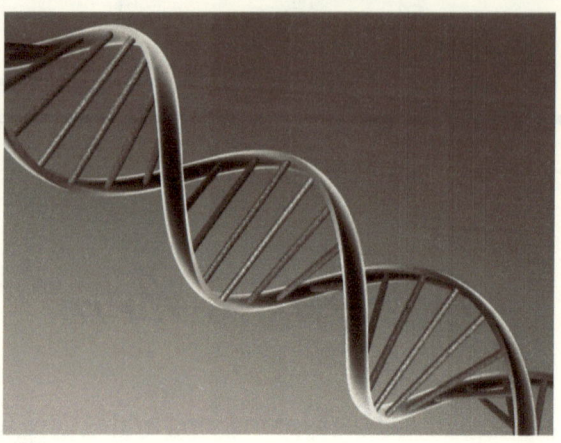

Now, people don't have to wonder about hair. They can simply add it and go. However, does that address the question of why synthetic hair is even needed in the first place? Without doubt men love long hair, but so do women. Long hair has been coveted by many, but a small portion of society has difficulty growing long hair. It is no one's fault. There are a number of factors that cause this to be a reality.

The most prevalent of factors is the genetic one. The most unique thing about black hair is that other ethnicities do not have the diversity that we do. Because hair is a complex of protein, a person's DNA directs the construct of hair itself. The more diverse the heritage means the more selection from which to construct the hair. Genetic diversity manifests itself as different hair textures and lengths. Therefore, this is why black hair is so variegated. Even the length of hair is directed by genes.

Lifestyle is another factor. The way you care for your hair starts with your diet. Hair length cannot be separated from the way you eat. There are products that can enhance your hair's appearance, but what about hair that is naturally beautiful? This may be harder to obtain, but the benefits outweigh the struggle.

We cannot forget the obvious factor of the Creator. Many times we women look in the mirror and think that that is where things end. We must assess our needs with the Lord in mind. If God created us with certain features, then we cannot think He made a mistake (Ps. 139)!

Hairlicious Is My Name

Hairlicious is my name
My hair affords my claim to fame
Please realize this
If you think I am unhappy
You think amiss

As a child my hair was not that wild
But to say I tamed it would be mild
The secret to my success would take just a while
In a matter of minutes I will turn your frown into a smile

The key is found in your food
Honestly, it will do your hair some good
Not to mention your heart loves vegetables too

CHAPTER 4

Truths about Hair

Now, in a perfect world your hair would reach its potential length. This is the reason Eve probably did maintain luxurious hair. She had no flatirons, blow-dryers, relaxer kits, straightening combs, etc. She ate from a bounty of vegetables and fruit. Meat was not an item of choice in the Garden of Eden from the beginning. This was not a problem since plants are more nutrient dense than meats. So what is the lesson we can learn from Eve? Granted she probably could not tell us much else because of her history, but there is truth behind her vegetarian diet. When she failed to eat vegetables then is when she had many problems that exceeded hair length.

1. Eve did not use products that damage hair. She did not have them. Flatirons, blow-dryers, curlers, and straightening combs emit great amounts of heat to style the hair. Such repetitive actions can dry one's hair, eventually robbing it off much-needed moisture. Hair that is dry is more susceptible to breaking than hair that is moisturized and well conditioned. Black hair needs moisture more than other cultures' hair.

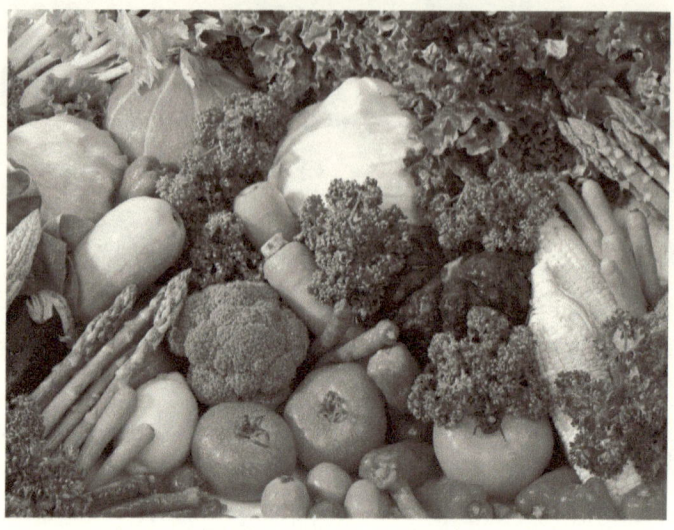

2. There is more to share about Eve's diet and hair. Increasing vegetables and fruit intake is helpful to support hair growth. Some people's diets are full of saturated fats and sugars. Isn't it ironic that your hair's growth may be as close as your mouth? Eve lived among a plethora of fruits and vegetables. It is no doubt that she made these the mainstay of her diet. Remember what got her in trouble in the first place?

   Flavonoids are antioxidants that are known to protect hair follicles while also encouraging hair growth. They are produced by plants. Carbohydrates and oils are not as dense with nutrients as plants are. Flavonoids can be found in apples, blueberries, and vegetables, just to name a few out of thousands of sources.

3. One memory that is prevalent about my childhood is the name-calling that little girls endured throughout primary school. It waned off with age, but the names are still in their memories and mine. I thought of such rudeness as specific to children until I heard a mother downgrading her daughter's hair. Thank the Lord for my mother. I must compel you to not allow others to curse your hair or even go along with them. The

power of death and life lies within the tongue. Negative words about appearance affect self-esteem.

4. Some herbs do deter baldness:

    Biotin promotes hair growth. It is found in brown rice, green peas, and sunflower seeds.

5. Keep the ends of your hair protected from the elements such as wind and rain by wrapping your hair ends. Wrapping or tying with silk cloth is usually sufficient. Because moisture is paramount for black hair, keeping hair away from the drying wind is a great help.

6. A relaxer/permanent is not permanent, but the damage to your cuticle layer is. The cuticle protects the hair. The greatest recourse for dry hair is to condition/moisturize the hair. If you don't want to relax your hair, then use other options for styling such as braiding or pressing.

7. Jojoba oil (*Simmondsia chinensis*) conditions the scalp or hair. It is one of the most dependable oils I know of from personal use. It also conditions the skin.

8. Hair vitamins are very helpful if you are unable to supplement your diet with ample fruits and vegetables. They can speed up the hair growth process, or at least that was my experience. Rome was not built in one day, so give your body time to enhance your hair.

9. Greasing or oiling your hair does not *make* your hair grow. Nutrition is what helps your hair to grow. Grease may give it a healthy sheen, but it does not contribute to the amino acid constitution of your hair. Actually, nothing *makes* hair grow.

10. Clip ends six to eight weeks apart.

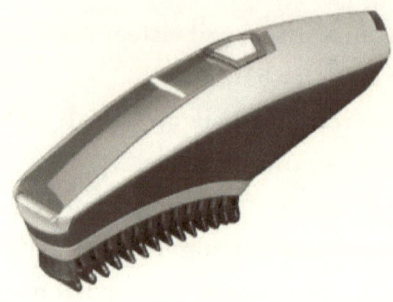

11. Use drying and styling agents as little as possible. Things such as hair paste, gels, and blow-dryers can dry your hair and may cause more drying than desired. Chemicals are not your hair's friends either.

12. On your days off from work or school, give your hair a day off. Let there it be a day when you don't use hair sprays, gels, flatirons, pressing combs, hot curlers, or anything electronic or unnatural.

13. You don't like stress, neither does your hair. Things like rubber bands placed too tightly and harsh brushing can stress your hair to breakage.

14. Wear a swimming cap while swimming or in the water to protect hair from chlorine and excess drying.

15. Don't forget that hair is for you and that you should not feel like a prisoner of your own hair. If you are tired of the same style for years, then seek to change it for yourself and don't feel like a prisoner of your own hairstyle. Seek professional help first if you are unsure about new products and then explore. I witnessed my family jump on a hair product craze, and I witnessed them fall out as soon as others reported their hair falling out from using this new product that promised hair to act so perfectly. Just a word of caution: if something sounds too good to be true . . .

16. Increasing your intake of essential fatty acids can help in hair growth. Essential fatty acids are fatty acids that are needed for health. They cannot be made naturally by the body; therefore, they must be added to the diet. Sources of essential fatty acids are fish oils, grape seed oil, and flaxseed oil.

17. Raw nuts and seeds benefit the hair and scalp.

18. Adding vitamin B complex to your diet will help improve the condition of your hair.

19. Do not brush your hair while it is wet.

20. Avoid foods that include raw eggs because of its containment of avidin. Avidin is a protein that binds to biotin.

21. Beware of the damage that emotional stress can cause. Emotional illness can be a thief of beautiful hair. Depression can cause loss of interest in even the most basic things, even hair maintenance. This includes washing hair, conditioning it, and combing it. Develop a support system ahead of time to help you in the stormy times of life to tend to your hair in case you can't. Just do this as a precaution. I do not believe depression sends you notices before it strikes.

22. Physical illness can cause you inability to tend to your hair. Have a support system already in place. You may have to establish a support fund to pay for services if you cannot find volunteers. This is another life instance that you may have no briefing concerning its arrival. Therefore, go ahead and set things in place just in case.

23. Avoid treating your hair roughly. This may mean brisk brushing to having unkempt braids.

24. Let your hair dry naturally after washing: skip the blow-dryer whenever possible.

25. Pat your hair dry.

26. Speak positive words concerning your hair even to your hair. Replace the misnomers with words of gratitude and love. Restore your happiness.

27. Avoid wearing braided hair for long periods. The tightness of the braid may cause a change in hair texture or hair loss itself.

When we learn that God so loved the word that He gave his only begotten Son, Jesus, we learn a lot. Primarily we learn those who believe in Him will have everlasting life and that love is what the world is in need of most assuredly. From cute little babies to the winos on the street corner, everyone needs love.

Love is expressed in action. Have you noticed how Valentine's Day is accompanied with expressions of love? Results ensue because of love. Either we love more or we love less. Sometimes a tinge of ambivalence settles in our hearts due to lack of true love. Therefore, we must be very careful to love children for who they are and not for what they possess. Parents are children's first source of love. To hear insults regularly about one's appearance from the parents is destructive. It has in some cases taught young kids how to dislike themselves. Hearing that their hair texture is the fault of one parent, expletives, and name-calling because of the hair's length or grade injures the self-esteem of a child. For some this stimulates memories, but to others this may have been the beginning of unforgiveness in their lives. Such memories must be addressed and not overlooked.

Comments abound in school and the work field concerning appearance. One soon learns that regardless of however the parent treated you, that parental love was still superlative to public love. This is where I learned that the prettiest girls could have my mom's compliments, but they did not have her love. I did. I lived a life unscathed of insults about my hair, but my friends did not. Sometimes my relatives would mention wishes or desires of having long hair. I could only wish for them, but now this is my way to share with others how they can help their hair reach its own potential.

Every person is different. Some people are tall while others are short. This is no surprise. Therefore, we should accept that some people will have long hair while it is normal that others will have shorter hair.

Each person's double helix is specific to the individual. Even so, there are ways to add extensions to the hair to get a desired look. The only question at this point is that considering the billions of dollars spent on hair, whether synthetic or not, how many dollars have been expended to repair that extensions only mask? Things such as insecurity and shame are only covered and not dealt with through adding hair to one's head.

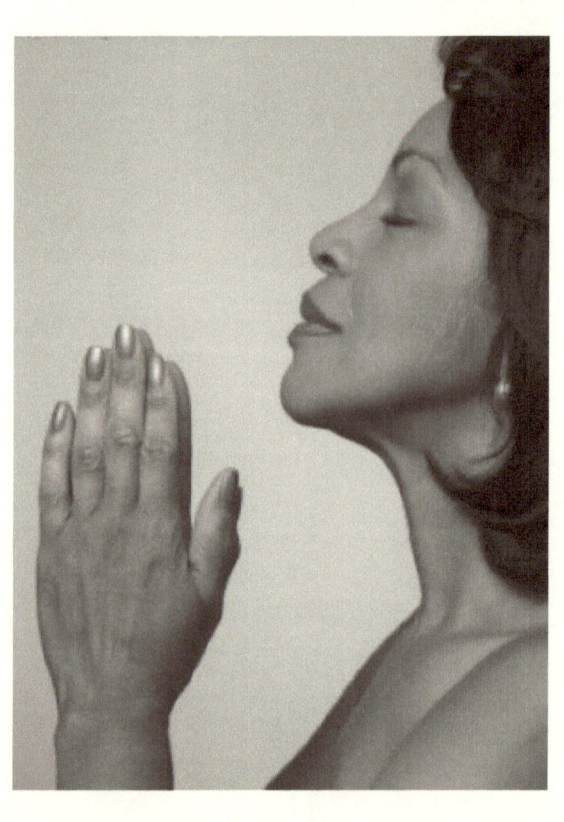

CHAPTER 5

Prayers

It would be entirely remiss of me to only bring attention to a matter without offering solutions. Therefore, here are some simple prayers that you can pray to receive forgiveness, experience healing, and promote change in the treatment of your fellow woman or man.

Forgiveness Prayer

Dear Father, you are worthy of all the praise. Please forgive me of all of my sins. I come before you regarding the matter of past hurts. First, I must address the instigator's place. Father, if hurt was placed on me because someone else did the same to the instigator, I ask you to heal them of their hurts that they would stop hurting others. Second, I lift up my situation to you. You know all of what has happened in the past, but it is having present effects on my peace. I will not let the same person who caused me injury to hinder me; therefore, I choose to forgive them. Erase the memories of pain if you will and teach me to let go of the pain. Teach me to let it go and live. In Jesus's name, amen.

Repentance Prayer

Dear Father, You are worthy of all praise. I confess that I have fallen short of the glory of God in life, and I acknowledge my need to repent of all my faults. Father, I declare as of today that I will live a changed life. I will live a life with other people's feelings in mind. Whether I agree or disagree with the choices of others, please help me to keep the hearts of others in plain view of my decision to voice my personal opinions. In Jesus's name, amen.

Healing Prayer

Dear Father,

You are worthy of all honor and acclaim. I confess that I have fallen short of the glory of God. Forgive me, Lord, of my sins and heal me of my hurt. It is my prayer that childhood memories would just remain so and that they do not hinder my daily walk in any way. Thank you for healing me for you are the Lord that heals me. In Jesus's name, amen.

There is no time like the present to invite you to receive Jesus Christ in your life because He shed his blood on the cross for our sins.

If you would like to invite Him, then confess that you are a sinner, pray to the Father to forgive you of your sins, tell Him that you repent of them. State that you believe Jesus to be Lord and Savior and that God raised Him from the dead on the third day.

Here is an example of a prayer for salvation:

Romans (10:9-10)

Dear Father,

I confess that I am a sinner. Forgive me of my sins because I do repent of them all. I believe that God raised you, Jesus, from the dead, and I do believe that Jesus is Lord and Savior. In Jesus's name I pray, amen.

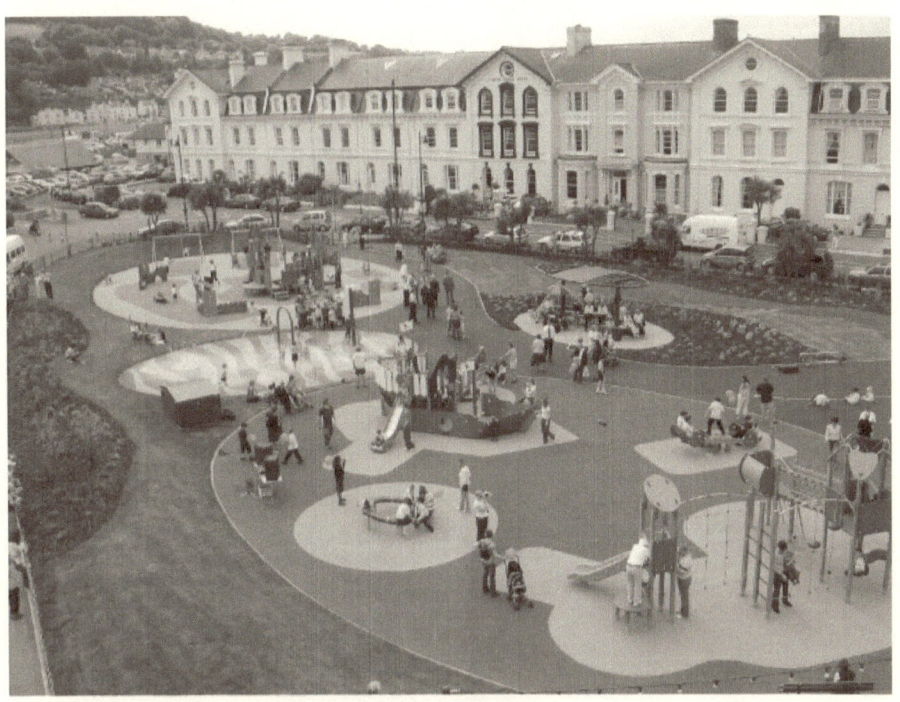

For the Children

My final thought concerns children:

Children are some of the most impressionable humans alive. There is a simple truth that must be remembered concerning children. An overwhelming majority of children base their self-esteem on their appearance. Because of this, criticisms can remain in their memories and linger past the formative years and contribute to low self-esteem during adulthood. Therefore, rather than affirming a child's looks, there is a more fruitful approach to helping. Focus on the character of a child. It can be developed as the child matures.

Bibliography

Balch, Phyllis A., CNC. *Prescription for Nutritional Healing*. New York: Avery, 2000.

"Hair." *Encyclopedia Britannica*. 4/14/2012. www.Britannica.com\ebchecked\topic 2518621.

Minirth, Frank, MD; Paul Meier, MD; and Stephen Arterburn M., eds. *The Complete Life Encyclopedia*. Nashville, 1995.

Taber's Cyclopedic Medical Dictionary. "Hair." 2009.

Willie Lynch Letter. Kashif Malik Hasfan-El. 4/14/2012. www.amazon.com/willie-lynch-letter-making-s\ave\dp\0948390530.

www.ingramcontent.com/pod-product-compliance
Lightning Source LLC
Chambersburg PA
CBHW050347290526
45785CB00006B/2664